Loving Someone with Dementia

Understanding, Coping, and Nurturing Through the Journey

Rachel J. Oles

All rights reserved. No part of this publication may be reproduced, distributed, or transmitted in any form or by any means, including photocopying, recording, or other electronic or mechanical methods, without the prior written permission of the publisher, except in the case of brief quotations embodied in critical reviews and certain other noncommercial uses permitted by copyright law.

Copyright © Rachel J. Oles, 2023.

Table of Contents

Chapter 1

<u>UNDERSTANDING DEMENTIA</u>

Dementia is a diverse and demanding disorder that affects millions of persons worldwide. This thorough book seeks to provide an in-depth overview of dementia, starting with the basics and moving to the numerous varieties, early signs and symptoms, and the degenerative nature of this disorder.

Dementia is not a single disease but an umbrella word used to describe a combination of symptoms and cognitive impairments that severely interfere with a person's ability to carry out daily activities. To grasp dementia better, let's break down its core features.

Dementia involves a spectrum of cognitive problems, including memory loss, decreased judgment, difficulties in problem-solving, and abnormalities in language and communication skills. These changes are often related to changes in brain function.

The Role of the Brain

To comprehend dementia, one must appreciate the role of the brain in cognitive functioning. The brain is a complicated organ made of billions of neurons that communicate through intricate networks. It is responsible for memory, reasoning, language, and other cognitive functions. Dementia affects these networks, resulting in the cognitive impairment seen in affected individuals.

Distinguishing Dementia from Normal Aging

Distinguishing dementia from the normal aging process is critical for both early diagnosis and the right therapy for cognitive abnormalities. It's vital to remember that aging is a natural and inevitable aspect of life, and experiencing certain cognitive changes as we age older is typical.

However, dementia indicates a medical state marked by more severe and progressive cognitive decline. In this talk, we will cover the fundamental differences between the two.

<u>Normal Cognitive Aging</u>

1. <u>Slower Information Processing:</u> It's natural for older folks to endure slower information processing and response times. This can manifest in tasks like decision-making, problem-solving, and reaction time. Dementia, on the other hand, results in major cognitive problems, including memory loss and decreased judgment.

2. <u>Mild Forgetfulness:</u> Occasional forgetfulness is a natural feature of aging. It

may involve misplacing keys, forgetting someone's name momentarily, or occasionally having difficulties recalling certain details. In dementia, memory loss is more severe and steadily worsens.

3. <u>Preserved Reasoning and Problem-Solving:</u> While older persons could experience some degree of cognitive deterioration, their capacity to reason and solve issues remains remarkably intact. Dementia, on the other hand, inhibits this higher-order cognitive functioning to a greater degree.

4. <u>Maintained Independence:</u> Older persons can typically continue living independently, managing their daily activities, and making wise judgments. Dementia generally leads to a loss of independence and the need for greater help.

5. <u>Consistent Social Engagement:</u> Normal aging doesn't usually result in social

disengagement or major changes in behavior. In dementia, personality changes and social isolation can be substantial.

6. <u>Steady Language abilities:</u> While older persons might occasionally struggle to find the correct term, they maintain steady language abilities overall. Dementia often leads to major language impairments.

7. <u>Awareness of Cognitive Changes:</u> Older persons are often aware of their cognitive changes and can compensate for them. Individuals with dementia typically lack an understanding of their cognitive limitations.

Dementia

1. <u>Progressive Cognitive deterioration:</u> Dementia is characterized by a progressive and persistent deterioration in cognitive function, generally starting with memory loss and spreading to a spectrum of cognitive and functional deficits.

2. <u>Significant Memory Loss:</u> While older folks might occasionally forget names or events, those with dementia exhibit profound and continuing memory loss, typically difficult to recall recent and prior events.

3. <u>Impaired Reasoning and Problem-Solving:</u> Dementia leads to marked difficulties in making judgments and solving problems. Simple decision-making gets extremely complex.

4. <u>Loss of Independence:</u> As dementia progresses, individuals lose their ability to carry out basic activities of daily living independently, including personal cleanliness, meal preparation, and medication administration.

5. <u>Personality and Behavioral Changes:</u> Dementia often results in personality changes, mood swings, and, in certain cases,

behavioral abnormalities like hostility and agitation.

6. <u>Social Withdrawal:</u> Individuals with dementia may retreat from social activities and connections due to communication issues and cognitive challenges.

7. <u>Severe Language Difficulties:</u> Language problems in dementia extend beyond sometimes searching for words. Conversations become increasingly disjointed and nonsensical.

8. <u>Lack of Insight:</u> One of the characteristic aspects of dementia is anosognosia, a lack of awareness of cognitive deficiencies. Individuals with dementia may not understand the severity of their memory and thinking impairments.

Common Types of Dementia

Dementia is a broad word, yet there are various different varieties, each with its unique traits and underlying reasons. Some of the most frequent kinds of dementia include:

Dementia is not a specific disease but rather an umbrella word that embraces a multitude of disorders, each with its individual characteristics, causes, and course. Understanding the many varieties of dementia is critical for accurate diagnosis, treatment, and care.

In this detailed discussion, we will look into some of the most common varieties of dementia, including Alzheimer's disease, vascular dementia, Lewy body dementia, frontotemporal dementia, and mixed dementia.

<u>Alzheimer's Disease</u>

Alzheimer's disease is the most widespread and widely recognized type of dementia, accounting for a major part of dementia cases. It is characterized by the buildup of aberrant protein deposits in the brain. These deposits include beta-amyloid plaques and tau tangles, which impede normal brain function.

<u>Key Features:</u>

- <u>Memory Impairment:</u> Alzheimer's often begins with short-term memory loss, gradually progressing to long-term memory loss.

- <u>Disorientation:</u> Individuals may feel bewildered about time, place, and people.

- <u>Language Difficulties:</u> Communication challenges and difficulty finding the correct words are prevalent.

- <u>Impaired Judgment:</u> Poor decision-making and judgment are seen.

- <u>Personality Changes:</u> Individuals may become irritated or apathetic.

- <u>Progressive Nature:</u> Alzheimer's disease is generally progressive, with discrete stages of cognitive impairment.

Vascular Dementia

Vascular dementia comes from diminished blood flow to the brain owing to vascular disorders, such as strokes or damaged blood arteries. It is frequently considered the second most common type of dementia.

Key Features:
- <u>Gradual Decline:</u> Cognitive decline can be abrupt and gradual, reflecting the impact of individual strokes.

- <u>Variability in Symptoms:</u> Symptoms can vary depending on the site of vascular injury.

- <u>Memory and Executive Function:</u> Impairments in memory and executive functioning are prevalent.

- <u>Emotional and Behavioral Changes:</u> Vascular dementia can lead to mood swings and emotional instability.

<u>Lewy Body Dementia</u>

Lewy body dementia is associated with aberrant protein deposits termed Lewy bodies in the brain. It shares certain similarities with both Alzheimer's disease and Parkinson's disease.

<u>Key Features:</u>

- <u>Visual Hallucinations:</u> Individuals often suffer visual hallucinations.

- <u>Fluctuating Cognitive Abilities:</u> Cognitive abilities might fluctuate during the day.

- <u>Parkinsonism:</u> Movement difficulties simulating Parkinson's disease, such as tremors and rigidity.
- <u>Attention and Alertness Fluctuations:</u> Alertness and attention can change, resulting in confusion and disorientation.

Frontotemporal Dementia

Frontotemporal dementia primarily affects the frontal and temporal lobes of the brain. It is quite infrequent but can be particularly tough to identify due to its variable clinical presentation.

Key Features:
- <u>Personality and Behavior Changes:</u> Individuals may display substantial personality and behavior changes.

- <u>Language Impairment:</u> Language impairments, including difficulty speaking and understanding language, are widespread.

- <u>Early-Onset:</u> Frontotemporal dementia commonly arises in adults under the age of 65.

- <u>Motor Symptoms:</u> Some variations of the disease include motor symptoms, such as muscle weakness.

Mixed Dementia

In some situations, individuals may exhibit characteristics of more than one type of dementia, which is referred to as mixed dementia. Mixed dementia might provide distinct diagnostic and management issues.

Key Features:

- <u>Multiple Pathologies:</u> Mixed dementia involves the presence of more than one form of dementia pathology, such as Alzheimer's and vascular dementia.

- <u>Varied Symptoms:</u> The symptoms of mixed dementia might vary and may involve a combination of cognitive, motor, and psychosocial aspects.

- <u>Complex Diagnosis:</u> Diagnosing mixed dementia frequently involves a complete investigation, including imaging and clinical tests.

Understanding the many varieties of dementia is vital for caregivers, healthcare workers, and researchers. Proper diagnosis and personalized care measures can dramatically enhance the quality of life for those living with dementia and their families. While each variety of dementia has its unique traits, they all have the common issue of cognitive decline and the need for compassionate care and support.

RECOGNIZING EARLY SIGNS AND SYMPTOMS

Dementia frequently starts with mild changes in cognitive function, making early recognition crucial. The early signs and symptoms of dementia might vary based on the individual type but may include:

Memory Loss

Memory loss is a defining symptom of dementia. Individuals may have difficulties recalling recent events, names, or significant details.

Confusion and Disorientation

Dementia can lead to confusion regarding time, place, and individuals. Individuals may become disoriented and find it tough to recognize familiar settings.

Difficulty with Language

A deterioration in linguistic skills is prevalent in dementia. This may show as problems finding the correct words, speaking coherently, or comprehending people.

Impaired Judgment and Decision-Making

Dementia can lead to impaired judgment and difficulties in making decisions. Individuals may make unusual choices, even placing their safety at risk.

Changes in Mood and Personality

Personality changes are often noted in dementia. Individuals may become irritable, agitated, or apathetic.

Decreased Problem-Solving Abilities

Dementia can hamper problem-solving skills, making tasks that were once regular more complex to execute.

Social Withdrawal
Dementia can lead to social disengagement and a lack of interest in previously appreciated activities.

Motor and Coordination Issues
In some varieties of dementia, such as Lewy body dementia, individuals may exhibit movement abnormalities similar to those seen in Parkinson's disease.

The Progressive Nature of Dementia
Dementia is often a progressive disorder, meaning that it worsens over time. Understanding this process is vital for caregivers and healthcare professionals to provide proper care and support.

STAGES OF DEMENTIA
Dementia is a progressive disorder that normally proceeds through various phases, each defined by specific deficits in cognitive, functional, and behavioral capacities. The

awareness of these stages is useful for caregivers, healthcare professionals, and families as it assists in planning and giving appropriate care and support.

While there isn't a universally agreed staging method for all types of dementia, a general framework can be applied to many cases. Here, we'll explore the typical phases of dementia:

Stage 1: Preclinical or Mild Cognitive Impairment (MCI)

This stage is typically not recognized as dementia, yet it indicates the early indicators of cognitive decline. Some patients with MCI may eventually progress to dementia, whereas others may not. The important elements of this stage include:

- <u>Subtle Memory Problems:</u> Individuals may have difficulties remembering recent events or specifics.

- <u>Mild Cognitive Changes:</u> The person can still manage routine activities and preserve independence.

- <u>Awareness of Changes:</u> Some persons at this stage are aware of their cognitive impairments, while others may not notice any issues.

Stage 2: Mild Dementia

This stage is frequently where most diagnoses arise, as the symptoms become more evident and interfere with daily life. Key characteristics of mild dementia include:

- <u>Memory Loss:</u> This is more evident than in the MCI stage and generally entails trouble recalling recent events, names, and locations.

- <u>Disorientation:</u> Individuals may get confused about the time, place, or identity of persons.

- <u>Language Difficulties:</u> Communication problems become increasingly apparent, with persons failing to find words and express themselves effectively.

- <u>Impaired Judgment:</u> Poor decision-making and judgment can be noted.
- <u>Personality Changes:</u> Some individuals may become irritated, worried, or withdrawn.

During this stage, persons can frequently carry out essential activities of daily living, such as personal cleanliness and meal preparation, although with some difficulty.

<u>Stage 3: Moderate Dementia</u>

Moderate dementia reflects a significant progression in cognitive decline and is characterized by:

-   <u>Severe Memory Impairment:</u> Both short-term and long-term memory losses are significant.

- <u>Increased Disorientation:</u> Individuals may not recognize familiar surroundings or faces.

-   <u>Communication Challenges:</u> Language challenges intensify, with persons having trouble comprehending others and expressing themselves.

- <u>Personality and Behavioral Changes:</u> Mood swings, anger, and hostility may become more apparent.

-   <u>Decreased Problem-Solving Abilities:</u> Individuals struggle with tasks that require planning and problem-solving.

- <u>Loss of Independence:</u> As cognitive capacities continue to diminish, persons may require assistance with most everyday activities.

Stage 4: Severe Dementia

In this advanced stage of dementia, persons become profoundly impaired, with a significant loss of cognitive and functional ability. Key aspects include:

- <u>Profound Memory Impairment:</u> Both short-term and long-term memory are significantly impacted.

- <u>Complete Disorientation:</u> Individuals may not recognize even close family members or their own reflection.

- <u>Limited Verbal Communication:</u> Many patients with severe dementia can no longer communicate or understand spoken language.

- <u>Severe Personality and Behavioral Changes:</u> Agitation, aggressiveness, and other behavioral disorders may become permanent.

- <u>Total Dependence:</u> Individuals require round-the-clock care for all daily activities, including feeding and toileting.

<u>Stage 5: End-Stage Dementia</u>

This ultimate stage is marked by the near-complete loss of cognitive, functional, and physical capacities. At this point:

- <u>Total Memory Loss:</u> Individuals no longer remember memories and have no remembrance of their history.

- <u>Inability to Communicate:</u> Verbal communication is lost, and non-verbal communication may be limited.

- <u>Complete Dependence:</u> Individuals are fully dependent on caretakers for all aspects of everyday life.

- <u>Physical Decline:</u> Physical health deteriorates, making the person susceptible to infections and other medical issues.

- <u>Loss of Mobility:</u> Individuals may become bedridden or require specific care to prevent pressure sores.

Caregivers and healthcare professionals must provide tailored care and support that addresses the particular needs and challenges of each person with dementia as they progress through these stages.

Chapter 2

COMMON MYTHS AND MISCONCEPTIONS

Myths and misconceptions regarding dementia are pervasive and can lead to misunderstandings, stigma, and insufficient treatment for persons living with dementia.

Myth 1: Dementia is a Normal Part of Aging

Fact: Dementia is not a natural result of aging. While it is true that the risk of having dementia grows with age, it is a medical illness that results from certain diseases or injury to the brain. Many older persons preserve their cognitive faculties and do not get dementia.

Myth 2: Dementia is All About Memory Loss

Fact: Memory loss is a common sign of dementia, but it is not the only one. Dementia can also influence judgment, problem-solving, language, conduct, and other cognitive skills. Different kinds of dementia may present with varying sets of symptoms.

Myth 3: Dementia is Inevitably Inherited

Fact: While there are some rare kinds of dementia with a strong hereditary component (e.g., familial Alzheimer's disease), most cases of dementia are not inherited. Advanced age and numerous lifestyle and environmental factors play a more significant influence in the development of most dementia kinds.

Myth 4: Dementia is Contagious

Fact: Dementia is not a contagious disease. It cannot be spread through physical contact, such as shaking hands or hugging, or by being in close proximity to someone with dementia. Dementia is a result of unique brain abnormalities that are not caused by germs or viruses.

Myth 5: Dementia is the Same as Alzheimer's Disease

Fact: Alzheimer's disease is just one type of dementia. Dementia is an umbrella word that incorporates different illnesses, including Alzheimer's, vascular dementia, Lewy body dementia, and frontotemporal dementia, among others. Each type of dementia has specific traits and underlying causes.

Myth 6: Only Elderly People Get Dementia

Fact: While dementia is more common in older folks, it can afflict individuals of all ages. Early-onset dementia can occur in persons in their 40s, 50s, or 60s. Age is a risk factor for dementia, however, it is not the sole determinant.

Myth 7: Dementia Can Be Cured

Fact: Currently, there is no cure for most cases of dementia. While some medications and actions can help control symptoms and reduce the progression of the condition, they do not eliminate the underlying reasons. Early diagnosis and effective care can make a considerable impact on a person's quality of life, but a total cure is not yet feasible.

Myth 8: People with Dementia Can't Understand or Communicate

Fact: People with dementia may understand and communicate, although their abilities may be impaired. It is vital to employ clear and straightforward language, non-verbal clues, and gestures to improve communication. Many individuals with dementia can still express emotions and wants.

Myth 9: Dementia is Always Accompanied by Aggressive Behavior

Fact: Aggressive conduct is not universal in dementia. While some individuals with dementia may exhibit agitation, hostility, or other behavioral abnormalities, not everyone with the diagnosis displays these characteristics. The experience of dementia varies greatly from person to person.

Myth 10: Nothing Can Be Done to Help Individuals with Dementia

Fact: There is much that can be done to support those with dementia. Therapeutic therapies, cognitive stimulation, and person-centered care techniques can improve the quality of life for those living with dementia. Additionally, assistance for caregivers and families is necessary to guarantee the well-being of all concerned.

Myth 11: All Dementia is the Same, and All Individuals with Dementia Are Alike

Fact: Dementia is a heterogeneous condition with distinct forms and presentations. Each individual's experience with dementia is unique. Understanding the precise form of dementia and the individual's history and preferences is vital for providing appropriate care and support.

Myth 12: People with Dementia Can't Live Independently

Fact: The ability of individuals with dementia to live independently varies on the stage and kind of dementia. In the early stages, many people can continue to live independently with sufficient care and safety measures. As the disease advances, additional support may be needed.

Myth 13: Individuals with Dementia Have No Quality of Life

Fact: People with dementia can experience a good quality of life if they receive sufficient care and support. Focusing on their residual talents, providing stimulating activities, and maintaining social relationships can boost their well-being and feelings of purpose.

Myth 14: Dementia is a Hopeless Condition

Fact: While dementia is a tough condition, there is hope and opportunity for individuals to live well with it. Support, understanding, and appropriate interventions can improve the quality of life for both those with dementia and their caregivers.

Myth 15: Dementia is Only About Loss

Fact: While dementia presents many obstacles and losses, it can also offer possibilities for personal growth, connection, and meaningful experiences.

Caregivers often find that their interactions with individuals with dementia deepen in beneficial ways.

Myth 16: Dementia is a Death Sentence

Fact: Dementia is a chronic disorder, although it is not necessarily a death sentence. Individuals with dementia can live for many years following diagnosis, especially with early intervention and proper care. The development of the disease varies greatly among individuals.

Myth 17: Dementia is Solely a Cognitive Condition

Fact: Dementia impacts more than cognition. It can also affect an individual's emotions, behavior, and physical health. Comprehensive care should address all elements of well-being.

Myth 18: There's Nothing You Can Do to Prevent Dementia

Fact: While certain risk factors for dementia, such as age and genetics, cannot be modified, there are modifiable risk factors. A healthy lifestyle, including regular exercise, a balanced diet, social involvement, and cognitive stimulation, can help lower the chance of acquiring dementia.

Myth 19: Dementia is Only About the Individual with the Diagnosis

Fact: Dementia has a tremendous impact on family and caregivers. Caregivers play a critical role in providing support and care, and they also need aid and support to overcome the obstacles of caregiving.

Myth 20: People with Dementia Should Be Isolated for Their Safety

Fact: While safety is necessary, social seclusion is not the answer. Individuals with dementia can benefit from social contact, mental stimulation, and physical activity. Caregivers should take measures to establish a safe but enriching environment.

Myth 21: Dementia Is a Solo Journey

Fact: Dementia is not a journey individuals must undergo alone. A solid support system, including family, friends, and healthcare experts, is vital. Collaborative care and emotional support from loved ones can considerably improve the quality of life for persons with dementia.

Myth 22: There's No Point in Seeking a Diagnosis

Fact: Early diagnosis of dementia is critical. While there is no cure, early intervention can help manage symptoms, enhance the individual's quality of life, and provide chances for care planning and legal and financial arrangements. A diagnosis also ensures that reversible sources of cognitive impairment are ruled out.

Myth 23: People with Dementia Can't Participate in Decision-Making

Fact: Individuals with dementia can and should be involved in decisions regarding their care and everyday lives, especially in the early stages. Their interests and values should be respected and taken into account while planning their care and making choices about living arrangements.

Myth 24: Individuals with Dementia Are Unaware of Their Surroundings

Fact: While individuals with advanced dementia may look unconscious of their surroundings, they can nevertheless experience emotions and respond to sensory cues. Creating a familiar and pleasant setting is vital for their well-being.

Myth 25: All Individuals with Dementia Are A Burden

Fact: Individuals with dementia continue to have value and can contribute to their families and communities. While caring can be tough, it can also be a rewarding and important experience.

Myth 26: Dementia Is Always a Steady Decline

Fact: The progression of dementia is not usually gradual. Some individuals experience periods of stability or even momentary improvement. Dementia trajectories can vary, and the rate of decline fluctuates among individuals.

Myth 27: Dementia Is Hopeless for Caregivers

Fact: While caregiving for someone with dementia is hard, caregivers can enjoy personal growth, resilience, and a deepened connection with their loved ones. Support and tools are available to help caregivers negotiate the hurdles.

Myth 28: Individuals with Dementia Should Be Institutionalized

Fact: Many individuals with dementia can live in familiar home situations or receive care in community-based settings. Residential care facilities or nursing homes are available, however, they should be chosen based on the individual's personal needs and preferences.

Myth 29: Dementia Means the End of Enjoyment

Fact: While some activities may become more problematic as dementia progresses, individuals can still experience moments of joy, connection, and meaningful engagement. Adapting activities to their skills can boost their quality of life.

Myth 30: Dementia Is a One-Size-Fits-All Condition

Fact: Dementia is exceedingly individual. Each person's experience is unique, and their treatment should be tailored to their personal needs, preferences, and degree of dementia. What works for one individual may not work for another.

Myth 31: Dementia Always Leads to Incoherence

Fact: While verbal impairments are frequent in dementia, not all individuals with the condition become incoherent. Many can still communicate effectively by gestures, expressions, and other non-verbal techniques.

Myth 32: Once Diagnosed, Nothing Can Be Done

Fact: While there is no cure, several interventions, therapies, and treatments can help control the symptoms and enhance the quality of life for those with dementia. Non-pharmacological treatments, including cognitive stimulation and creative therapies, are increasingly regarded as useful.

Myth 33: There's No Point in Researching Dementia

Fact: Dementia research continues to make advances. Understanding the causes, risk factors, and potential therapies is crucial. Participating in clinical trials can contribute to developments in dementia care and potentially lead to breakthroughs.

Myth 34: Dementia Is a Death Sentence

Fact: Dementia is a chronic disorder, and individuals can live with it for many years. Some persons maintain an excellent quality of life for an extended period, especially with early diagnosis and appropriate care.

Myth 35: Dementia Is a Western Problem

Fact: Dementia is a global issue, not isolated to Western countries. It affects people from varied ethnic origins and places globally. Cultural competence is vital in delivering dementia care that respects cultural norms and values.

Addressing myths and misconceptions about dementia is vital for creating understanding, empathy, and effective treatment. Dementia impacts individuals and their families on a physical, emotional, and social level, and a more accurate understanding of the condition helps encourage a caring and inclusive approach to dementia care.

By refuting these stereotypes, we can work toward eliminating stigma and ensuring individuals with dementia can live with dignity and quality of life.

Chapter 3

<u>DIAGNOSIS</u>

The diagnosis procedure of dementia is a critical and often challenging journey that comprises a number of exams and evaluations to confirm the presence of cognitive impairment and determine the underlying cause.

This procedure is vital to offer individuals and their families a clear awareness of the illness and guide proper care and planning. Let's discuss the essential components of the diagnosis procedure of dementia:

<u>Recognizing Cognitive Changes</u>

The diagnostic procedure often begins when individuals, family members, or friends notice cognitive abnormalities or behavioral adjustments in an individual.

These changes may be minor at first but grow more pronounced or persistent with time. Common early signs of cognitive decline include:

1. <u>Memory Lapses:</u> Frequent forgetting, especially remembering recent events, appointments, or discussions.

2. <u>Difficulties in Communication:</u> Struggling to find the correct words, frequent pauses in talking, or difficulties following conversations.

3. <u>Challenges in Daily Activities:</u> Struggling to accomplish routine chores, such as managing finances, preparing meals, or following directions.

4. <u>Personality Changes:</u> Noticeable modifications in emotional responses, conduct, or personality features. This may

include increased irritation, mood fluctuations, or social disengagement.

Seeking Medical Evaluation

Once cognitive abnormalities are found, the affected people or their loved ones often seek a medical evaluation to determine the cause of these changes and to rule out reversible or treatable diseases. The evaluation procedure frequently begins by making an appointment with a healthcare expert, such as a primary care physician, geriatrician, or neurologist. The medical examination contains numerous key components:

1. Medical History

The healthcare provider will acquire a detailed medical history. This includes information regarding the individual's past and present medical conditions, medications, family medical history, and any recent events that may be pertinent to the cognitive changes.

2. Physical Examination

A complete physical examination is undertaken to assess the individual's overall health and to rule out any physical disorders that could be contributing to the cognitive abnormalities. This checkup may include checking for indicators of infections, metabolic disorders, or other medical concerns.

3. Cognitive Tests

Standardized cognitive tests are conducted to examine many elements of cognitive performance. These exams help establish a baseline of cognitive ability and examine memory, attention, language, problem-solving, and other cognitive domains. Common cognitive tests include the Mini-Mental State Examination (MMSE), the Montreal Cognitive Assessment (MoCA), and others.

4. Neuroimaging

To visualize the brain's structure and identify any abnormalities, neuroimaging examinations such as magnetic resonance imaging (MRI) and computed tomography (CT) scans are often conducted. These pictures can reveal evidence of brain atrophy, the existence of lesions, or other anatomical alterations linked with dementia.

5. Blood Tests

Blood tests may be undertaken to screen out possibly reversible causes of cognitive impairment. These tests can uncover problems including vitamin shortages, thyroid issues, or metabolic disorders that may influence cognitive performance.

Diagnosis Confirmation

Once the assessments are finished, the healthcare provider makes an official diagnosis, confirming the presence of dementia. This diagnosis is often based on criteria from established diagnostic standards, such as the Diagnostic and Statistical Manual of Mental Disorders (DSM-5) or the International Classification of Diseases (ICD-10/11).

The diagnosis includes specifying the type of dementia, such as:

- Alzheimer's Disease: The most prevalent form of dementia, characterized by the deposition of beta-amyloid plaques and tau protein tangles in the brain.

- Vascular Dementia: Often caused by a history of stroke or other cerebrovascular illnesses that affect the brain's blood vessels.

- Lewy Body Dementia: Characterized by the presence of aberrant protein deposits (Lewy bodies) in the brain, leading to cognitive and motor symptoms.

- <u>Frontotemporal Dementia:</u> A less common type of dementia affecting the frontal and temporal lobes of the brain, leading to changes in behavior, personality, and language.

- <u>Mixed Dementia:</u> In cases where different kinds of dementia are present, a diagnosis of mixed dementia is given.

The Role of Neuropsychological Assessment

In some circumstances, a full neuropsychological assessment may be recommended to give a more in-depth evaluation of cognitive ability. This evaluation, often conducted by a neuropsychologist, contains a battery of tests and assessments that explore multiple cognitive domains in detail.

Neuropsychological evaluations can provide a more precise knowledge of the individual's cognitive strengths and deficiencies, aiding in the diagnostic process and therapy planning.

Challenges in the Diagnostic Process

The diagnostic process of dementia can be challenging due to several factors:

- <u>Variability in Symptoms:</u> Dementia symptoms can vary widely between individuals, and they may overlap with symptoms of other medical diseases.

- <u>Stigma and Denial:</u> Individuals and their families may be reluctant to obtain a diagnosis due to the stigma associated with dementia and the fear of confirming cognitive deterioration.

- <u>Differential Diagnosis:</u> Distinguishing between distinct varieties of dementia can be complicated, as many symptoms are common among various forms of the disorder.

- <u>Co-Existing Conditions:</u> Dementia can co-exist with other medical situations, making it crucial to rule out other contributory causes.

The Importance of Early Diagnosis

An early and accurate diagnosis of dementia is critical for various reasons:

- <u>Treatment and Intervention:</u> Early diagnosis can lead to timely intervention, allowing individuals to receive suitable treatments and support services that can help manage symptoms and delay the progression of the disease.

- <u>Planning for the Future:</u> It enables individuals and their families to plan for the future, make decisions about care, and establish legal and financial arrangements.

- <u>Reversible Causes:</u> Some cognitive abnormalities may be attributable to curable or reversible causes. Identifying these factors early can result in effective therapy and potential improvement.

- <u>Clinical Trials and Research:</u> Early diagnosis permits patients to participate in clinical trials and research aimed at increasing our understanding of dementia and identifying new therapies.

The diagnostic procedure of dementia is a complex but crucial trip to confirm the presence of cognitive impairment and determine the underlying cause.

While it can be emotionally taxing, early identification opens the way to appropriate care, treatment, and planning, ultimately enhancing the quality of life for those living with dementia and their family. It is crucial for individuals, families, and healthcare providers to interact throughout this process to guarantee the greatest potential outcomes.

Chapter 4

<u>NAVIGATING A LIFE-ALTERING REVELATION</u>

Receiving a diagnosis of dementia is a life-altering experience for both the people affected and their loved ones. This comprehensive discussion delves into the various aspects of the dementia diagnosis, including the experience of receiving and processing the diagnosis, communicating it to the affected individual, seeking professional guidance and support, and the emotional responses that accompany this critical revelation.

<u>Receiving and Processing the Diagnosis</u>

Receiving a dementia diagnosis is a key time, frequently riddled with confusion, dread, and uncertainty. It's crucial to understand how the process occurs and how individuals and their families may manage this hard phase.

Emotional Impact of the Diagnosis

Shock and Denial: The initial reaction to a dementia diagnosis might often be one of shock and denial. Individuals and their families may find it hard to accept the reality of cognitive decline.

Grief and Loss: The diagnosis signifies a huge loss, not just for the individual but also for their loved ones. This loss might elicit feelings of grief and despair.

Uncertainty About the Future: The unknown course of dementia might induce concern about what lies ahead. Planning for the future can become intimidating.

Stigma and Social Isolation: The stigma associated with dementia can contribute to social isolation, as individuals and their families may withdraw from social activities due to fear of judgment.

<u>Communicating the Diagnosis to the Loved One</u>

Effectively communicating a dementia diagnosis to the affected individual is a delicate and vital phase in the process. Open and empathetic communication is crucial for offering emotional support and increasing understanding.

<u>Preparing for the Conversation</u>

<u>Choosing the Right Setting:</u> Selecting a comfortable and private place for the discussion is key. Avoid distractions and ensure there's adequate time for questioning and emotional processing.

<u>Having Support Present:</u> Having a trusted family member, friend, or healthcare professional present throughout the chat can provide emotional support and assist in resolving questions.

The Conversation

Using Clear and Simple Language: It's vital to use basic, straightforward language to express the diagnosis, avoiding medical jargon that could be confusing.

Providing Information: Share information regarding the type of dementia, its progression, and potential treatment choices. Encourage inquiries and conversations.

Expressing Empathy: Communicate your love, support, and empathy for the impacted individual. Acknowledge their emotions and concerns.

Offering Hope: Emphasize that life doesn't stop with a dementia diagnosis and that there are ways to preserve a good quality of life, even as the condition advances.

Emotional Responses

Shock and Denial: The affected individual may initially respond with disbelief or denial, which is a natural defense strategy.

Grief and Sadness: As the reality of the diagnosis sets in, the person may experience grief and sadness for the losses connected with dementia.

Anger and Frustration: Feelings of anger and frustration are frequent, directed towards the circumstances, the diagnosis, or even toward loved ones.

Fear and Anxiety: Fear of the unknown and anxiety about the future can be overwhelming. This is a crucial emotional response to address.

Resilience and Acceptance: Over time, some individuals come to terms with the diagnosis and display extraordinary resilience and adaptability.

<u>Seeking Professional Guidance and Support</u>

A dementia diagnosis not only the sufferer but also their caretakers and family. Seeking expert assistance and support is vital for achieving the greatest possible care and quality of life.

<u>Healthcare Professionals</u>

<u>Specialized Healthcare Teams:</u> Access to neurologists, geriatricians, neuropsychologists, and dementia experts can give a complete approach to dementia care.

<u>Medication and Treatment Options:</u> Healthcare experts can administer medications and offer treatments to manage symptoms and reduce the progression of the condition.

Support Services

Caregiver help Groups: Caregivers often seek help and direction in managing the challenges of dementia care. Support groups can offer important support.

In-Home Care: Professional caregivers can provide in-home support with daily activities, allowing individuals to remain in a familiar environment.

Adult Day Programs: These programs offer a safe and stimulating environment for adults with dementia while offering relief for caretakers.

Legal and Financial Planning

Legal Documents: Preparing legal documents such as power of attorney, living will, and guardianship is crucial to guarantee that the individual's desires are respected as the disease develops.

<u>Financial Planning:</u> Planning for the expense of care, managing assets, and accessing available financial resources is vital for the long-term financial well-being of the affected individual.

Emotional Responses to the Diagnosis

Emotions play a crucial role in the journey following a dementia diagnosis, both for the individual and their loved ones. Understanding and managing these emotions is vital for delivering thorough care and support.

Grief and Loss

- <u>Anticipatory Grief:</u> Grief can begin even before a severe cognitive decline occurs as individuals and their families anticipate the losses that dementia will bring.

- <u>Multiple Losses:</u> Dementia involves a sequence of losses, including loss of independence, loss of memories, and finally, the loss of the person's previous self.

Fear and Anxiety

- <u>Fear of the Future:</u> The unpredictable aspect of dementia typically leads to dread about what lies ahead, including potential impairments in cognitive and physical ability.

- <u>Concern About Caregiving:</u> Caregivers often suffer concern about their ability to provide essential care and the consequences of caregiving on their own well-being.

Anger and Frustration

- <u>Anger at the Disease:</u> Individuals and their loved ones may experience anger and frustration towards the disease itself, as it robs them of their quality of life.

- <u>Social Isolation:</u> The stigma connected with dementia can contribute to sentiments of anger and frustration over the lack of understanding and support from society.

Sadness and Depression

- <u>Persistent Sadness:</u> The continual problems of dementia care can contribute to persistent feelings of sadness and, in some circumstances, depression.

- <u>Social Withdrawal:</u> Both individuals with dementia and their caretakers may withdraw from social activities due to grief and a sense of isolation.

<u>Resilience and Acceptance</u>

- <u>Adaptive Coping:</u> Over time, some persons and their caregivers display extraordinary tenacity and adaptability, discovering methods to live well with dementia.

- <u>Acceptance of the Situation:</u> Acceptance of the diagnosis and its problems is an important emotional response that can lead to a more positive view.

Navigating the diagnosis and its emotional impact is an important phase in the dementia journey, and it lays the way for better care, quality of life, and the well-being of both those with dementia and their caregivers.

Chapter 5

<u>THE CAREGIVER'S ROLE</u>

Caring for someone with dementia is a difficult and very sympathetic role that brings both obstacles and pleasures. In this extensive exploration, we will delve into the multifaceted aspects of the caregiver's role in dementia care, including the emotional journey, the delicate balance between self-care and caregiving, the critical legal and financial considerations, and the importance of building a robust support network.

<u>The Caregiver's Role</u>

The caregiver's position in dementia care is one that needs love, patience, and a strong commitment to the well-being of the individual with dementia. Understanding the obligations, challenges, and rewards of this profession is vital for giving the best care possible.

<u>Responsibilities of a Caregiver</u>

1. <u>Assistance with Daily Activities:</u> Caregivers often support patients with dementia in activities of daily living, such as bathing, clothing, grooming, and meal preparation.

2. <u>Medication Management:</u> Ensuring that the individual takes their prescribed medications on time and as advised is a key element of caregiving.

3. <u>Emotional Support:</u> Providing emotional support and companionship to alleviate feelings of loneliness and anxiety in the individual with dementia.

4. <u>Safety and Supervision:</u> Ensuring the safety of the individual by supervising them and establishing safety measures to prevent accidents or wandering.

5. <u>Communication:</u> Facilitating clear and effective communication, which becomes increasingly challenging as dementia progresses.

6. <u>Crisis Management:</u> Handling tough conditions, such as agitation or disorientation, in a calm and sympathetic manner.

Challenges of the Caregiver's Role

<u>Emotional Toll:</u> Caregiving may be emotionally exhausting, often leading to feelings of stress, guilt, and grief as caregivers observe the demise of their loved one.

<u>Physical Demands:</u> The physical demands of caregiving, especially in the case of individuals with advanced dementia, can be demanding.

Social Isolation: Caregivers may face social isolation as they commit significant time and energy to their role.

Financial Strain: The cost of dementia care, including medical bills and long-term care, can represent a major financial hardship.

Lack of Sleep: Caregivers often endure sleep interruptions, leading to their own health difficulties.

Rewards of the Caregiver's Role

Despite the hardships, caring can also be deeply rewarding:

Sense of Fulfillment: Caregivers frequently find a tremendous sense of fulfillment and purpose in caring for their loved ones.

Quality Time: Spending quality time with the individual and developing cherished memories can be immensely gratifying.

<u>Bonding:</u> Caregiving can deepen the link between the caregiver and the individual with dementia.

<u>Personal Growth:</u> Many caregivers discover inner resilience, adaptation, and personal growth throughout their journey.

The Caregiver's Emotional Journey

The emotional journey of a caregiver in dementia care is distinguished by a range of feelings that vary over time. Understanding and managing these emotions is vital for preserving the caregiver's well-being and providing high-quality care.

Initial Emotions

<u>Shock and Denial:</u> Caregivers may first experience shock and denial upon obtaining the dementia diagnosis. This phase

generally comprises denial and the hope that the cognitive alterations are transient.

Grief and Loss: Grief is a frequent emotional response, both for the individual with dementia and their caretakers. Caregivers may grieve the gradual loss of the person they previously knew.

Emotions During Caregiving

Stress and Anxiety: As caregiving obligations increase, caregivers typically experience stress and anxiety. Concerns for the individual's well-being, and safety, and managing the everyday demands of care can be overwhelming.

Guilt: Caregivers may fight with emotions of guilt, especially when they need to make difficult decisions or take breaks from caregiving.

<u>Anger and Frustration:</u> The persistent nature of dementia care can rise to sentiments of anger and frustration. These feelings may be directed against the disease, the situation, or even the individual with dementia.

<u>Melancholy and Depression:</u> Persistent melancholy and, in certain situations, depression can arise as caregivers cope with the constant demands of caring.

<u>Weariness and Burnout:</u> The physical and emotional demands of caregiving can lead to caregiver weariness and, in some circumstances, burnout.

Emotions as Dementia Progresses

<u>Acceptance and Adaptation:</u> Over time, some caregivers acquire a level of acceptance and adapt to the reality of dementia care. This phase frequently entails

learning to find joy and contentment in the current moment.

<u>Compassion and Empathy:</u> Caregivers typically develop profound compassion and empathy as they experience the fragility and needs of the individual with dementia.

Balancing Self-Care and Caregiving

Balancing self-care with caregiving is a critical component of providing excellent care while maintaining the caregiver's own well-being. Neglecting self-care can lead to caregiver burnout and impair the quality of care delivered.

The Importance of Self-Care

Caregivers often put their own needs and well-being on the back burner. However, self-care is necessary for various reasons:

<u>Maintaining Physical Health:</u> Prioritizing self-care helps caregivers stay physically healthy, ensuring they have the energy and stamina to provide care.

<u>Preserving Mental Health:</u> Self-care supports the caregiver's mental health, lowering stress, anxiety, and symptoms of depression.

<u>Preventing Burnout:</u> Burnout is a big danger for caregivers. Self-care techniques can help minimize caregiver burnout, which can be detrimental to both the caregiver and the individual with dementia.

<u>Enhancing the Quality of Care:</u> Caregivers who prioritize self-care are better suited to offer high-quality care and maintain a positive, patient-centered attitude.

<u>Legal and Financial Considerations</u>

Caring for someone with dementia also includes addressing crucial legal and financial matters to ensure the individual's well-being and plan for the future. Failing to address these concerns can lead to complications and challenges down the road.

<u>Legal Considerations</u>

<u>Power of Attorney:</u> Appointing someone to act as the individual's power of attorney for healthcare and financial choices is vital. This guarantees that their wishes are upheld when they are no longer able to make decisions.

<u>Living Will:</u> A living will describe the individual's healthcare wishes, notably addressing end-of-life decisions. It provides direction for medical decisions when the individual cannot articulate their wishes.

Guardianship: In circumstances when a person with dementia is no longer able to make decisions and has not appointed a power of attorney, guardianship may be necessary to make legal decisions on their behalf.

Estate Planning: Addressing estate planning, including wills and trusts, is vital to guarantee that the individual's assets and property are managed according to their wishes.

Long-Term Care Planning: Planning for long-term care, including decisions concerning residential care facilities, is an important legal factor.

Financial Considerations

Budget and Expenses: Caregivers must set a budget and monitor expenses linked to dementia care. This includes fees for drugs, medical appointments, in-home care, and residential care if necessary.

<u>Insurance:</u> Reviewing insurance policies, especially health insurance and long-term care insurance, is necessary to assure coverage for dementia-related expenses.

<u>Social Services and Benefits:</u> Investigating available social services and benefits, such as Medicaid or veterans' benefits, might provide financial support for dementia care.

<u>Legal Assistance:</u> Consulting with an attorney who specializes in elder law and estate planning can provide useful guidance for resolving financial concerns.

BUILDING A SUPPORT NETWORK

Building a solid support network is vital for caregivers in dementia care. Caregiving is not a solo path, and having a network of support can provide emotional, practical, and respite assistance.

<u>Family and Friends</u>

Family members and friends can play a vital part in the caregiver's support network. They can offer emotional support, share caregiving chores, and provide respite care when needed.

<u>Support Groups</u>

Support groups designed for dementia caregivers provide a secure and empathic venue to share experiences, obtain advice, and find understanding. These organizations might be in-person or online.

<u>Professional Caregivers</u>

Professional caregivers and in-home care services can aid with every day caring responsibilities and provide relief for family caregivers. These services can minimize the stress on the primary caregiver.

<u>Therapists and Counselors</u>

Therapists and counselors can provide emotional support, coping skills, and assistance for managing the emotional problems of caregiving.

Community Resources

Community resources, such as adult day programs, respite care, and memory care facilities, can offer practical support and social involvement for those with dementia.

Legal and Financial Advisors

Legal and financial consultants can offer guidance on legal and financial problems, helping caregivers make educated decisions.

The caregiver's involvement in dementia care is a profound and complex journey, distinguished by duties, challenges, and rewards. Understanding the emotional journey, the necessity of self-care, legal and financial considerations, and the benefit of a robust support network is crucial for delivering the best possible care to those with dementia and sustaining the caregiver's well-being.

Caregivers are unsung heroes in the field of dementia care, and their dedication and compassion make a huge difference in the lives of individuals they care for.

Chapter 6

PROVIDING PHYSICAL CARE

Caring for individuals with dementia involves a particular combination of abilities and a grasp of their fluctuating needs as the condition progresses.

Ensuring Safety and Comfort at Home

Creating a safe and comfortable home environment is vital for those with dementia. Safety precautions help prevent accidents and ensure that the individual feels secure and at peace in their surroundings. Here are crucial measures for ensuring safety and comfort at home:

1. Minimize Hazards

Identify and mitigate potential dangers in the home environment, including:

- Removing tripping risks such as loose rugs and clutter.
- Installing handrails and grab bars in the restroom and other high-risk areas.
- Ensuring good illumination to lessen the danger of falls and confusion.
- Securing sharp things, hazardous substances, and potentially harmful goods.

2. Wandering Prevention

Individuals with dementia may roam, posing safety issues. Implement the following precautions:

- Install door alarms and locks to prevent straying without restricting freedom.
- Use GPS tracking devices or bracelets to locate the person if they do wander.
- Consider motion sensor alarms in critical parts of the home.

3. Medication Safety

Pharmaceutical management is vital to avoid pharmaceutical errors. Ensure safety by:

- Organizing drugs in a pill organizer or blister packs.
- Supervising drug delivery to prevent accidental overdose.
- Regularly dispose of expired or unused drugs.

4. Monitoring Temperature

Individuals with dementia may struggle to maintain body temperature. Maintain comfort by:

- Adjusting room temperatures to a comfortable level.
- Dressing the individual in proper clothing for the season.
- Providing fans or space warmers if necessary.

5. Personalized Spaces

Create a familiar and welcoming environment by:

- Displaying family photos and souvenirs.
- Using familiar furniture and arrangements to reduce confusion.
- Providing a comfy chair or location for leisure and activity.

6. Mealtime Safety

Safety during meals is vital to prevent choking and guarantee sufficient nutrition. Safeguard mealtime by:

- Offering tiny, manageable servings of meals.
- Cutting food into bite-sized pieces.
- Monitoring the individual during meals to prevent choking.

Managing Daily Activities (Eating, Bathing, Dressing, Medication)

As dementia progresses, managing daily activities becomes increasingly challenging. Caregivers must change their approach to ensure the individual's needs are satisfied while safeguarding their dignity and liberty.

1. Eating and Nutrition

Nutrition is a key element of care for patients with dementia. To promote healthy eating and ensure appropriate nutrition:

- Provide a balanced diet with a range of foods.
- Offer familiar, favored meals to encourage eating.
- Use adaptable utensils and plates if needed.
- Monitor for signs of choking and modify the diet as necessary.
- Ensure proper hydration by providing water regularly.

2. Bathing and Personal Hygiene

Bathing and personal hygiene can be distressing for those with dementia. To make this process more comfortable:

- Maintain a consistent bathing practice to reduce anxiety.
- Use warm water and a moderate approach to make the experience more enjoyable.
- Provide verbal cues and step-by-step directions to guide the individual.
- Ensure privacy and dignity by utilizing shower curtains or screens.

3. Dressing and Grooming

Dressing and grooming can be tough due to cognitive and physical changes. Simplify the procedure by:

- Offering alternatives to the individual to offer a sensation of control.
- Laying out garments in the order they should be put on.

- Using garments with easy fastening, such as Velcro or elastic bands.
- Being patient and allowing extra time for dressing and grooming.

4. Medication Management

Managing drugs for adults with dementia is vital to their health and well-being. Ensure medication management by:

- Using a pill organizer or blister packs to sort and deliver medications.
- Offering visual or audible cues to remind the user to take their prescription.
- Documenting drug schedules and any negative effects.

<u>Coping with Incontinence</u>

Incontinence is a typical concern in dementia care and can be stressful for both the client and the caregiver. Effective techniques to manage incontinence include:

1. Maintain a Routine

Establish a regular toileting plan to prevent accidents. Encourage the individual to use the bathroom at consistent intervals, such as after meals or before bedtime.

2. Provide Supportive Products

Use incontinence items such as adult diapers or pads to manage accidents. Ensure they are comfortable and fit properly.

3. Maintain Hydration

Proper hydration is vital to prevent urinary tract infections. Ensure the individual consumes enough fluids but monitor for overhydration in the evening to reduce nighttime mishaps.

4. Promote Hygiene

Emphasize proper hygiene practices, including thorough cleaning and replacement of incontinence products. This is vital for reducing skin irritation and infections.

5. Consult a Healthcare Professional

If incontinence is persistent or worsening, visit a healthcare practitioner to treat any underlying medical disorders or infections that may be contributing to the problem.

<u>Dealing with Mobility Issues</u>

As dementia progresses, individuals may experience mobility challenges, making it challenging for them to walk securely and comfortably. Here are techniques for coping with mobility concerns in dementia care:

1. Fall Prevention

Falls are a substantial risk for those with dementia. Prevent falls by:

- Keeping paths clear and free from impediments.
- Installing handrails and grab bars in essential areas, such as the restroom.

- Using non-slip mats on slick areas.

2. Assistive Devices

Mobility aids can promote safety and independence. Consider the use of:

- Walkers or canes to provide help whilst walking.
- Wheelchairs for those with limited mobility.
- Bed rails to assist with getting in and out of bed safely.

3. Transfer Techniques

Assisting adults with dementia in transferring from one posture to another involves specialized strategies. Caregivers should be taught safe transfer methods to avoid injury to both the caregiver and the individual.

4. Exercise and Physical Activity

Encourage physical activity to maintain strength and mobility. Simple exercises and activities, such as light walks or chair exercises, can help.

5. Engage Occupational and Physical Therapists

Consult with occupational and physical therapists who specialize in dementia care. They can provide specific techniques and exercises to increase mobility and reduce fall risks.

Providing physical care for those with dementia needs careful preparation, sensitivity, and a deep awareness of the unique problems associated with the condition.

Ensuring safety and comfort at home, managing daily routines, living with incontinence, and resolving mobility concerns are critical parts of dementia care.

Caregivers play a critical role in enhancing the quality of life for those with dementia, and their dedication is invaluable in delivering the best possible care.

Chapter 7

<u>NURTURING EMOTIONAL WELL-BEING</u>

Emotional well-being is a vital part of caring for those with dementia. Understanding and supporting their emotional needs is vital for boosting their quality of life and general well-being.

This includes understanding their emotional experience, tactics for reducing anxiety and agitation, establishing emotional connections, and the crucial role of music, art, and reminiscence therapy.

<u>Understanding the Emotional Experience of the Loved One</u>

Understanding the emotional experience of individuals with dementia is the foundation for delivering good care and support.

Dementia can bring forth a spectrum of complicated emotions, which evolve as the condition worsens. Key components in understanding the emotional experience include:

1. Emotional States

- <u>Anxiety:</u> Individuals with dementia often experience heightened anxiety owing to disorientation and trouble interpreting their environment. This might lead to restlessness and agitation.

- <u>Depression:</u> Feelings of melancholy and despair are prevalent, coming from a sense of loss and the problems of dementia.

- <u>Frustration and Agitation:</u> Difficulty in communication and executing daily chores might result in frustration and agitation.

- <u>Fear and Paranoia:</u> Individuals may become scared owing to their failure to perceive their environment, leading to paranoia and suspicion.

- <u>Isolation:</u> Social isolation can be emotionally distressing, as individuals may withdraw from social engagements owing to the stigma associated with dementia.

- <u>Emotional Resilience:</u> Despite the challenges, some individuals with dementia display emotional resilience and flexibility, finding moments of serenity and delight.

2. Communication Challenges

Understanding the emotional experience is hindered by communication issues. As dementia progresses, individuals may fail to communicate their emotions verbally. Observing nonverbal signs, body language, and changes in behavior is vital to determining their emotional condition.

3. Emotional Triggers

Identifying emotional triggers might help caregivers provide a more supportive atmosphere. Triggers may include changes in habit, unusual situations, or sensory overload.

<u>Strategies for Reducing Anxiety and Agitation</u>

Reducing anxiety and agitation is vital for promoting emotional well-being in those with dementia. Caregivers might apply many techniques to address these emotional issues effectively:

1. Establish a Consistent Routine

A consistent daily routine can create a sense of comfort and lessen anxiety. Consistency in meal times, activities, and rest intervals might help people feel more at peace.

2. Create a Calming Environment

Minimize potential stressors by providing a peaceful and pleasant environment. This may involve:

- Reducing noise levels.
- Using soft, natural lighting.
- Decorating using familiar and comforting items.
- Employing relaxing smells, such as lavender.

3. Engage in Relaxation Techniques

Simple relaxation exercises can help ease anxiety and agitation. Techniques include deep breathing techniques, progressive muscle relaxation, and mindfulness meditation.

4. Validation and Reassurance

Validation is a powerful tool in dementia care. Acknowledge the individual's feelings, even if they don't fit with reality. Reassure them and provide comfort.

5. Distract and Redirect

When individuals grow irritated, distracting and redirecting their attention to a new activity or topic might be useful in resolving the situation.

6. Sensory Stimulation

Sensory activities, such as mild massage, tactile objects, and calming music, can help folks relax and reduce anxiety.

7. Medication and Medical Intervention

In some circumstances, medical intervention may be necessary to address acute anxiety and agitation. Medications recommended by a healthcare expert should be taken as a last option and strictly monitored.

Fostering Emotional Connection

Maintaining emotional ties with individuals with dementia is crucial for their well-being. Building and cultivating these ties may be both tough and rewarding. Strategies for creating emotional relationships include:

1. Effective Communication

Using basic and plain language helps boost communication. Maintain eye contact, use gestures, and offer positive reinforcement to make the individual feel understood.

2. Active Listening

Listening attentively and patiently to the individual's remarks, even if they appear senseless, displays respect and empathy.

3. Engaging in Shared Activities

Participating in things that the individual enjoys can create positive shared experiences. This may involve hobbies, puzzles, or listening to music.

4. Touch and Physical Affection

Gentle touch, such as holding hands or providing hugs, can provide comfort and emotional connection.

5. Storytelling and Reminiscence

Encouraging the individual to tell tales and reminisce about the past helps develop emotional bonds. Create opportunities for people to share their life experiences.

6. Show Unconditional Love

Individuals with dementia may exhibit problematic behaviors, but providing unconditional love and patience is vital for preserving emotional ties.

The Role of Music, Art, and Reminiscence Therapy

Music, art, and reminiscence therapy offer important channels for cultivating emotional well-being in adults with dementia. These therapies draw into creativity and memory to engage the individual and produce positive emotional responses:

1. Music Therapy

- <u>Benefits:</u> Music has a tremendous impact on emotions and memory. It can elicit nostalgia, boost mood, and reduce anxiety and agitation.

- <u>Methods:</u> Play familiar songs, sing together and utilize music to stimulate reminiscences. Consider employing personalized playlists and musical instruments.

2. Art Therapy

- <u>Benefits:</u> Art therapy gives a creative outlet for self-expression and emotional release. It can boost self-esteem and cognitive function.

- <u>Methods:</u> Provide art supplies and encourage the individual to draw, paint, or participate in other artistic pursuits.

3. Reminiscence Therapy

- <u>Benefits:</u> Reminiscence therapy involves discussing and reflecting on prior events. It can boost memory, increase self-esteem, and develop emotional bonds.

- <u>Methods:</u> Create a memory box with souvenirs, look at photo albums or engage in guided reminiscing sessions.

Nurturing emotional well-being in adults with dementia is a varied and caring task. Understanding their emotional experience, applying tactics to minimize anxiety and agitation, building emotional connections, and harnessing the power of music, art, and reminiscence therapy can boost their quality of life and general well-being.

Caregivers and healthcare professionals play a vital role in fostering a supportive and emotionally enriching environment for individuals with dementia, ensuring that they enjoy comfort, connection, and moments of joy throughout their journey.

Chapter 8

COPING WITH PROGRESSION AND LOSS

Coping with the progression of dementia and the losses it involves is a very emotional and demanding journey for individuals with dementia, their families, and caregivers.

Recognizing Stages of Dementia

Dementia is a progressive disorder with multiple stages, each accompanied by its own set of obstacles and changes. Recognizing these stages is crucial for understanding what to expect and how to adapt care and support. The most prevalent paradigm for understanding dementia stages is:

1. Early Stage (Mild Dementia)
- **Characteristics:** In the early stage, individuals may experience modest memory

lapses, such as forgetting names or appointments. They can often do daily duties independently.

- **Challenges:** Coping with the dread and frustration that memory lapses bring. Concerns about cognitive changes may lead to worry and uncertainty.

2. Middle Stage (Moderate Dementia)

- **Characteristics:** As dementia progresses, persons in the middle stage suffer more pronounced cognitive problems. They may become disoriented, have difficulties communicating, and require support with daily activities.

- **Challenges:** Caregivers must adapt to increased care demands, control mood swings, and manage behavioral changes, such as agitation or hostility. Grief for the person's prior capabilities may also be widespread.

3. Late Stage (Severe Dementia)

- **<u>Characteristics:</u>** The late stage is distinguished by considerable cognitive and functional impairment. Individuals may lose the ability to communicate, recognize loved ones, or conduct basic duties.

- **<u>Challenges:</u>** Caregivers must provide intensive care, addressing mobility difficulties, incontinence, and the danger of infections. Grief and sadness may be intense as individuals lose their sense of self.

4. End-of-Life Stage

- **<u>Characteristics:</u>** The end-of-life period entails a considerable deterioration in physical and cognitive functions, frequently with minimal reaction.

- **<u>Obstacles:</u>** Caregivers and family members face the emotional and practical obstacles of delivering palliative care and assuring comfort during this final phase.

<u>Coping with Memory Loss and Personality Changes</u>

Coping with memory loss and personality changes is a fundamental element of dementia care. As the condition worsens, individuals may display behaviors and symptoms that can be emotionally distressing for both the person with dementia and their caretakers. Strategies for coping with these changes include:

1. Empathy and Patience

Approaching memory loss and personality changes with empathy and tolerance helps promote a more positive and supportive atmosphere.

2. Validation and Redirection

Validation tactics, such as accepting the individual's sentiments even if they don't fit with reality, can lessen suffering. Redirection, where the individual's focus is directed to a different topic or activity, can be beneficial in addressing problematic behaviors.

3. Structured Routines

Establishing established daily routines can provide a sense of consistency and comfort, minimizing anxiety and confusion.

4. Adaptive Communication

Adapting communication tactics, such as using basic and clear language and visual clues, can promote understanding and minimize frustration.

5. Engagement in Meaningful Activities

Engaging the individual in meaningful activities that correspond with their interests and capabilities can increase their feeling of well-being and lessen emotional distress.

Grief and Anticipatory Grief

Grief is a vital element of dementia care for both the individual with dementia and their loved ones. Anticipatory grief, in particular, is a sort of grieving experienced before the real loss occurs. Grief and anticipatory grief can be triggered by:

1. Loss of Abilities

As individuals with dementia lose their cognitive and functional abilities, loved ones may grieve the steady decline and the person they once knew.

2. Changing Relationships

Dementia can affect relationships, leading to feelings of loss and grief for the way the connection previously was.

3. Loss of Future Plans

The onset of dementia may lead to the abandoning of future aspirations and dreams, leading to anticipatory grief.

4. End-of-Life Considerations

The end-of-life stage of dementia is accompanied by great pain and loss as loved ones prepare for the inevitable.

Coping with loss and anticipating grieving entails seeking assistance, knowing that these emotions are normal, and allowing oneself to grieve in a healthy way. This may include counseling, support groups, and self-care.

Preparing for End-of-Life Care

End-of-life care in dementia is a challenging and emotionally fraught phase of the journey. Preparing for end-of-life care entails several essential considerations:

1. Advance Care Planning

- <u>Advance Directives:</u> Individuals with dementia should write advance directives, including living wills and durable power of attorney for healthcare, to specify their end-of-life preferences and choose a healthcare proxy.

- <u>Do-Not-Resuscitate (DNR) Orders:</u> Discuss the propriety of DNR orders with a healthcare practitioner.

2. Palliative Care and Hospice

- <u>Palliative Care:</u> Palliative care focuses on enhancing the quality of life by managing symptoms and giving emotional and psychological support. Consider integrating palliative care into the individual's treatment plan.

- <u>Hospice Care:</u> Hospice care is acceptable in the late stages of dementia, offering comfort and support to patients and their families during the end-of-life period.

3. Emotional Support

End-of-life care can be emotionally stressful. Seek emotional help through counseling, support groups, or spiritual guidance to traverse this phase.

4. Legal and Financial Matters

Ensure that legal and financial matters, such as estate planning and the administration of assets, are in order. Consulting with an attorney who specializes in elder law might be useful.

5. Comfort and Quality of Life

Focus on providing comfort and boosting the individual's quality of life throughout this period. Consider pain management, emotional support, and assuring the presence of loved ones.

6. Family Discussions

Open and honest discussions with family members regarding end-of-life care decisions are crucial to ensure that everyone is on the same page and that the individual's desires are respected.

Coping with progression and loss in dementia care is a profound and difficult journey, distinguished by the recognition of dementia phases, the management of memory loss and personality changes, the experience of sadness and anticipatory grief, and the preparation for end-of-life care.

Caregivers, families, and individuals with dementia should approach this journey with empathy, patience, and a sincere dedication to giving the best available care and support.

By recognizing the various parts of this emotional and hard process, individuals with dementia can experience comfort and dignity, and their loved ones can navigate the path with compassion and grace.

Chapter 9

SELF-CARE STRATEGIES FOR CAREGIVERS

Caring for someone with dementia is a difficult and emotionally challenging duty. While it can be deeply satisfying, it's crucial for caregivers to prioritize their own well-being and practice self-care.

The Importance of Self-Care for Caregivers

Caregivers play a key role in the lives of those with dementia. They provide critical support, sympathy, and love. However, the duties of caregiving can take a toll on the caregiver's physical and emotional health. It's vital to know that taking care of oneself is not a luxury but a need.

When caregivers exercise self-care, they are better positioned to provide high-quality care, reduce stress, and avoid caregiver burnout. Here are several strong reasons for caregivers to prioritize self-care:

1. <u>Physical Well-Being:</u> Self-care activities such as regular exercise, healthy nutrition, and adequate sleep are vital for preserving physical health. Caregivers who are healthy can provide better care.

2. <u>Emotional Resilience:</u> Self-care practices assist caregivers in managing the emotional obstacles of caregiving, such as sadness, frustration, and stress. Emotional well-being is vital for sustaining long-term care.

3. <u>Reducing Stress:</u> Caregiving can be stressful. Practicing self-care decreases stress and helps caregivers remain patient and composed.

4. <u>Preventing Burnout:</u> Caregiver burnout is a substantial concern when self-care is

neglected. Burnout can lead to physical and mental weariness, ultimately impacting the quality of treatment offered.

5. <u>Enhancing Care Quality:</u> Caregivers who prioritize self-care can deliver greater quality care and maintain a patient-centered approach.

Self-Care Strategies for Caregivers

Effective self-care tactics comprise a spectrum of physical, emotional, and social practices. Caregivers might consider implementing these self-care measures into their regular routines:

Physical Self-Care

1. <u>Exercise:</u> Engage in regular physical activity, such as walking, yoga, or swimming. Exercise not only promotes physical health but also decreases stress and boosts happiness.

2. <u>Nutrition:</u> Maintain a balanced diet with plenty of fruits, vegetables, and whole grains. Proper eating helps overall health and energy levels.

3. <u>Sleep:</u> Ensure adequate sleep. Create a sleep-friendly environment, set a nightly routine, and prioritize rest.

4. <u>Medical Check-Ups:</u> Attend regular medical check-ups to monitor your personal health. This is especially crucial for caregivers who may overlook their own well-being.

5. <u>Relaxation:</u> Incorporate relaxation techniques such as deep breathing, meditation, or progressive muscle relaxation into your regular routine to reduce stress.

<u>Emotional Self-Care</u>

1. <u>Seek Emotional Support:</u> Connect with friends, family members, or support groups. Talking about your feelings and experiences can be beneficial.

2. <u>Set Boundaries:</u> Establish boundaries to prevent caregiver burnout. It's alright to say no or ask for help when you need it.

3. <u>Journaling:</u> Maintain a caregiving journal to express your thoughts and feelings. This can provide a good outlet for your emotions.

4. <u>Therapy and Counseling:</u> Consider seeing a therapist or counselor who specializes in caregiver concerns. Professional support can offer direction and coping skills.

5. <u>Mindfulness:</u> Practice mindfulness practices to stay present in the moment and minimize worry and stress.

Social Self-Care

1. <u>Maintain Social Connections:</u> Nurture your social connections and engage in activities you like. Socializing with friends and loved ones provides a break from caregiving and helps maintain a support network.

2. <u>Respite Care:</u> Utilize respite care services to take breaks from caregiving. Respite care helps you to recharge and respond to your own needs.

3. <u>Support Groups:</u> Join caregiver support groups, whether in-person or online. These groups offer empathy, advice, and a sense of connection with others who understand your struggles.

4. <u>Ask for Help:</u> Don't hesitate to ask for help when you need it. Enlist family members or friends to assist with caregiving tasks or to provide emotional support.

Practical Self-Care

1. <u>Time Management:</u> Implement effective time management tactics to ensure you have time for yourself. Scheduling regular breaks and sticking to a pattern can assist.

2. <u>Hobbies and Interests:</u> Continue pursuing your hobbies and interests. Engaging in activities you enjoy can bring a sense of fulfillment.

3. <u>Respite Care:</u> Consider respite care services that provide temporary relief from caregiving responsibilities. This can be invaluable for self-care.

4. <u>Legal and Financial Planning:</u> Address legal and financial problems, including power of attorney, wills, and financial planning. Planning for the future helps alleviate stress and ensure your loved one's well-being.

Resources for Caregiver Support

There are various resources available to encourage caregivers in their self-care efforts:

1. <u>Caregiver Support Organizations:</u> Organizations like the Alzheimer's Association and the Family Caregiver Alliance offer resources, information, and support for caregivers.

2. <u>Local Support Services:</u> Many areas offer local support services, including respite care, support groups, and adult day programs.

3. <u>Online Communities:</u> Online forums and social media groups provide a platform for caregivers to interact, exchange stories, and obtain advice.

4. <u>Books and Publications:</u> A variety of books and publications are dedicated to caregiving and self-care for caregivers.

5. <u>Healthcare experts:</u> Consult with healthcare experts, social workers, and therapists who can provide assistance on self-care and support services.

Caring for someone with dementia is a noble and humane task, but it can also be emotionally exhausting. Prioritizing self-care is not a sign of neglect but a demonstration of self-compassion and a commitment to provide the best possible care.

By combining physical, emotional, social, and practical self-care practices into your routine, you may preserve your well-being, minimize stress, and continue to be a source of love and support for your loved one with dementia.

Chapter 10

<u>FINDING SUPPORT AND RESOURCES</u>

Caring for someone with dementia is a demanding and often emotionally challenging journey. Caregivers require a solid support structure and access to resources to offer the best possible care and maintain their own well-being.

<u>Local and Online Support Groups</u>

Support groups are essential sources of emotional aid, practical advice, and a feeling of community for caregivers. Whether you prefer in-person meetings or the convenience of online forums, these organizations give a safe area to share experiences and interact with others who understand the challenges of dementia care.

Local Support Groups

Local support groups offer face-to-face interaction and can be especially helpful for caregivers who desire direct personal connections with others in their region. Here's how to identify and benefit from local support groups:

1. <u>Search Online:</u> Start by looking online for support groups in your region. Organizations like the Alzheimer's Association often conduct local meetings and can help you identify nearby organizations.

2. <u>Community Centers:</u> Check with community centers, elder centers, and religious organizations, as they may organize support groups for caregivers.

3. <u>Hospitals and Healthcare professionals:</u> Hospitals, memory care clinics, and healthcare professionals sometimes offer or

recommend local support groups for caregivers.

4. <u>Ask for Referrals:</u> Your loved one's healthcare staff, such as their primary care physician or neurologist, may be able to recommend you to local support groups.

5. <u>Visit Meetings:</u> Attend a local support group meeting to see if it's a suitable fit for your requirements. You can also obtain information and resources during these meetings.

Online Support Groups

Online support groups offer flexibility and the opportunity to interact with caregivers from across the world. Consider the following when seeking support online:

1. <u>Dedicated Websites:</u> Numerous websites and forums are specifically established for caretakers of individuals with dementia.

Popular options include the Alzheimer's Association message boards, AgingCare.com, and the Alzheimer's Society's online community.

2. Social Media: Social media platforms, such as Facebook and Reddit, feature various caregiver support groups. Search for relevant organizations and request to join ones that fit your needs.

3. Privacy and Privacy: Online support groups allow you to engage with a level of privacy if you want not to share personal information. You can engage in debates and ask questions without disclosing your name.

4. Availability 24/7: Online support groups are available at any time, making it ideal for caregivers with hectic schedules or those who require assistance outside of traditional meeting hours.

5. <u>Resource Sharing:</u> Online communities regularly exchange resources, articles, and helpful information relating to dementia care, making it a wonderful source of information.

Respite Care and Professional Help

Respite care and professional support are vital for caregivers to prevent burnout, maintain their health, and ensure that their loved one with dementia receives the best possible care. These services offer brief relief from caring chores and access to specialist expertise.

Respite Care

Respite care gives short-term reprieve to caregivers by allowing someone else to take over caregiving chores for a predetermined period. Here's how to access respite care:

1. <u>Local Respite Programs:</u> Investigate local programs or facilities that offer respite care

services. These may include adult day programs, assisted living facilities, or home care organizations.

2. Government Assistance: Many government programs, such as Medicaid and the National Family Caregiver Support Program, may cover respite care expenditures for qualifying individuals.

3. Nonprofit Organizations: Charitable organizations and foundations may provide financial support or connect caregivers with respite care services.

4. Veterans' Benefits: If your loved one is a veteran, examine the benefits available through the U.S. Department of Veterans Affairs (VA), providing respite care options.

5. Ask for Help: Don't hesitate to seek out friends and family members for temporary caregiving assistance, even if it's just for a few hours.

Professional Help

Professional aid can enhance the quality of care offered to individuals with dementia and alleviate some of the caregiving strain. Consider the following professional services:

1. <u>In-Home Care:</u> In-home care services provide skilled caregivers who can aid with daily routines, such as bathing, dressing, and meal preparation, right in the comfort of your loved one's home.

2. <u>Memory Care Facilities:</u> Memory care facilities are specialized care environments designed to fulfill the unique needs of individuals with dementia. They offer complete care, safety measures, and structured activities.

3. <u>Hiring a Geriatric Care Manager:</u> A geriatric care manager is a professional who can analyze your loved one's needs, design a

care plan, and arrange services, all while offering expert direction.

4. <u>Occupational and Physical Therapy:</u> Occupational and physical therapists can work with adults with dementia to increase mobility, retain independence, and address unique issues.

5. <u>Counseling and Psychotherapy:</u> Mental health specialists can provide counseling to caregivers, helping them cope with the emotional problems of caregiving.

6. <u>Legal and Financial Advisors:</u> Consulting with legal and financial professionals can assist in making key decisions, such as setting up powers of attorney, estate planning, and managing financial matters.

Palliative and Hospice Care

Palliative and hospice care services focus on enhancing the comfort and quality of life for patients with severe dementia, as well as giving support to their relatives. These services are offered to persons who require end-of-life care.

Palliative Care

Palliative care attempts to alleviate pain and enhance the quality of life for patients with dementia. It can be integrated at any stage of the disease and includes:

1. <u>Symptom Management:</u> Palliative care providers focus on controlling the symptoms of dementia, such as pain, agitation, and discomfort.

2. <u>Emotional Support:</u> Caregivers and family members receive emotional support to help them overcome the obstacles of severe dementia.

3. <u>Discussion and Decision-Making:</u> Palliative care teams enable open discussion

about care decisions and the individual's preferences.

4. <u>Holistic Care:</u> Care comprises the physical, emotional, social, and spiritual well-being of the individual.

5. <u>Care Coordination:</u> Palliative care providers interact with the individual's healthcare team to ensure comprehensive care.

6. <u>Home-Based Care:</u> Palliative care can be offered in numerous places, including at home, in hospitals, or in hospice centers.

Hospice Care

Hospice care is a specialized style of care developed for those with a terminal illness or at the end stage of dementia. Key features of hospice treatment include:

1. <u>Comfort-Centered Care:</u> The focus is on boosting comfort, pain control, and emotional support in the last stages of dementia.

2. <u>Pain and Symptom Management:</u> Hospice care specialists are experts in managing pain, discomfort, and uncomfortable symptoms.

3. <u>Emotional and Spiritual care:</u> Hospice staff offer emotional and spiritual care for both the individual and their family members.

4. <u>Quality of Life:</u> Hospice care seeks to ensure the best possible quality of life during the end-of-life phase.

5. <u>Caregiver Assistance:</u> Hospice programs extend assistance to caregivers, aiding them in coping with the emotional issues of end-of-life care.

6. <u>Grief and Bereavement assistance:</u> Hospice services offer bereavement assistance to family members and caregivers after the individual's passing.

Accessing Palliative and Hospice Care

Access to palliative and hospice care services often requires a healthcare provider's referral. You can commence the process by discussing the individual's situation with their primary care physician, who can connect you with suitable resources.

Many hospice and palliative care providers offer complete help, including setting up home-based care, which can be very advantageous for patients with late dementia who prefer to remain in familiar surroundings.

Community Resources for Dementia Care

Community resources for dementia care cover a wide range of services and support networks available to persons and caregivers in local communities. These resources can enhance the quality of care, provide educational opportunities, and offer aid in different aspects of dementia care.

1. <u>Local Dementia Care groups:</u> Many localities have groups dedicated to dementia care and assistance. These organizations can give information, resources, and guidance on local services.

2. <u>Dementia-Friendly Communities:</u> Some communities are actively working to become dementia-friendly by offering training to businesses, community organizations, and first responders to better understand and help individuals with dementia.

3. <u>Adult Day Programs:</u> Adult day programs provide a safe and exciting setting for adults with dementia. These programs offer planned activities, social connections, and respite for caregivers.

4. <u>Transportation Services:</u> Transportation services can help individuals with dementia access medical appointments and community activities. Some localities offer specific transportation choices for persons with cognitive disabilities.

5. <u>Legal and Financial Assistance:</u> Local groups, such as elder law attorneys, can provide legal and financial counsel for caregivers and individuals with dementia.

6. <u>Home Modification Programs:</u> Some communities offer home modification programs that can promote safety and accessibility for individuals with dementia, such as installing handrails, ramps, and safety measures.

7. <u>Educational Workshops and Seminars:</u> Look for local workshops, seminars, and educational activities pertaining to dementia care. These can provide helpful information and techniques for caretakers.

8. <u>Community Caregiver Support Programs:</u> Many communities have caregiver support programs that offer services like counseling, respite care, and education for caregivers.

9. <u>Volunteer Programs:</u> Volunteer organizations often provide vital support to individuals with dementia and their caretakers. Volunteers can aid with companionship, transportation, and everyday tasks.

10. <u>Art and Music Therapy Programs:</u> Some communities provide art and music therapy programs specifically developed for individuals with dementia. These programs

can increase emotional well-being and cognitive stimulation.

Finding assistance and resources for dementia care is vital for caregivers and individuals alike. Whether you're searching local or online support groups, respite care, palliative and hospice care, or community services, there is a plethora of aid available.

The road of caring for someone with dementia is tough, but with access to these resources and support networks, you may traverse the path with greater confidence, knowledge, and emotional fortitude. Remember that you are not alone, and there is a wide network of caregivers and specialists eager to assist you in providing the best possible care for your loved one with dementia.

www.ingramcontent.com/pod-product-compliance
Lightning Source LLC
Chambersburg PA
CBHW050825260726
48660CB00004B/1607